# Emotional Self-Care for Black Women

Discover How to Raise Self-Esteem,
Silence Inner Critic, Overcome Anxiety,
and Master Emotions for Lasting
Healing and Confidence

ALINA ROBERTSON

# Disclaimer

The information provided in this book is for educational and informational purposes only. It is not intended to be a substitute for professional medical advice, diagnosis, or treatment. Always seek the advice of your physician or other qualified health provider with any questions you may have regarding a medical condition.

The author and publisher of this book make no representations or warranties regarding the accuracy, applicability, or completeness of the contents of this book. The author and publisher disclaim any liabilities or loss in connection with the use of this book.

The reader assumes full responsibility for the use of the information provided in this book. The author and publisher shall not be held liable for any damages or losses arising from the use or misuse of the information contained herein.

# TABLE OF CONTENTS

# Introduction

In today's fast-paced world, where demands on our time and energy seem never-ending, prioritizing emotional well-being is essential for overall health and happiness. For Black women, navigating the complexities of life can often feel like an uphill battle, compounded by systemic injustices, societal pressures, and cultural expectations. In this book, we delve into the critical topic of emotional self-care specifically tailored to the experiences and needs of women.

## Understanding the Importance of Emotional Self-Care

Emotional self-care is not merely an indulgence but a vital aspect of maintaining holistic health. It involves recognizing, honoring, and addressing our emotional needs to foster resilience, inner peace, and self-compassion. By prioritizing emotional well-being, Black women can better navigate the various challenges they encounter, whether personal, professional, or societal.

## Acknowledging Unique Challenges Faced by Black Women

women face a myriad of unique challenges that can take a toll on their emotional health. From navigating systemic racism and discrimination to managing intersecting identities, such as race, gender, and socioeconomic status, the burdens can feel overwhelming. Moreover, societal expectations often place unrealistic demands on Black women to be strong, resilient, and self-sacrificing, leaving little room for vulnerability or self-care. Recognizing and acknowledging these challenges is the first step toward crafting effective strategies for emotional resilience and well-being.

# Cultivating Self-Awareness

Self-awareness is the foundation of emotional intelligence and an essential component of emotional self-care. It involves developing a deep understanding of our thoughts, feelings, behaviors, and triggers. By cultivating self-awareness, Black women can gain insight into their inner world, recognize patterns of thought and behavior, and make conscious choices that support their well-being. In this section, we explore two key aspects of cultivating self-awareness: exploring personal emotions and triggers, and identifying and challenging negative thought patterns.

**Exploring Personal Emotions and Triggers**
One of the first steps in cultivating self-awareness is to explore our personal emotions and understand what triggers them. For Black women, emotions can be complex and multifaceted, often influenced by both

individual experiences and broader social factors. Taking the time to acknowledge and validate our emotions, without judgment or suppression, is crucial for emotional well-being.

To explore our emotions, we can start by practicing mindfulness and tuning into our physical sensations, thoughts, and feelings in the present moment. This can be as simple as taking a few deep breaths, closing our eyes, and bringing our attention inward. By observing our emotions without attachment or reaction, we can begin to develop a deeper understanding of our inner landscape.

Additionally, journaling can be a powerful tool for exploring emotions. Writing down our thoughts and feelings allows us to externalize them, gain perspective, and identify recurring patterns or themes. We can ask ourselves questions such as "What am I feeling right now?" and "What events or situations triggered these emotions?" By identifying the specific triggers that elicit emotional responses, we can better prepare ourselves to navigate similar situations in the future.

Furthermore, seeking support from trusted friends, family members, or mental health professionals can provide valuable insights and validation. Sharing our emotions with others allows us to feel heard, understood, and supported, fostering a sense of connection and belonging.

## Identifying and Challenging Negative Thought Patterns

In addition to exploring our emotions, cultivating self-awareness involves identifying and challenging negative thought patterns that contribute to emotional distress. Negative thought patterns, also known as cognitive distortions, are habitual ways of thinking that are irrational, unhelpful, and often inaccurate. Common cognitive distortions include black-and-white thinking, catastrophizing, and personalization.

To identify negative thought patterns, we can practice self-reflection and introspection. Paying attention to our internal dialogue and noticing recurring themes or messages can help us identify distorted thinking patterns. For example, we may catch ourselves engaging in all-or-nothing thinking, such as believing that if we make a mistake, we are a total failure.

Once we have identified negative thought patterns, we can begin to challenge them by examining the evidence and considering alternative perspectives. This involves asking ourselves questions such as "Is this thought based on facts or assumptions?" and "What evidence do I have to support or refute this thought?" By critically evaluating our thoughts, we can develop more balanced and realistic interpretations of ourselves and our experiences.

Furthermore, practicing self-compassion and self-validation is essential for challenging negative thought patterns. Instead of harshly criticizing ourselves for our thoughts and feelings, we can adopt a compassionate and understanding attitude. We can remind ourselves that it is natural to experience a range of emotions and that our worth is not determined by our thoughts or perceived shortcomings.

Cultivating self-awareness is a powerful practice that empowers women to understand themselves on a deeper level, navigate their emotions with greater ease, and make choices that align with their values and priorities. By exploring personal emotions and triggers, and identifying and challenging negative thought patterns, women can develop the resilience and self-compassion needed to thrive in the face of life's challenges.

# Nurturing Self-Compassion

Self-compassion is a fundamental aspect of emotional self-care, especially for women who often face societal pressures, stereotypes, and systemic injustices that can erode their sense of self-worth and belonging. Nurturing self-compassion involves treating oneself with kindness, understanding, and acceptance, regardless of external circumstances. In this section, we explore two key strategies for nurturing self-compassion: embracing and celebrating Black identity and beauty, and practicing forgiveness and letting go of guilt.

**Embracing and Celebrating Black Identity and Beauty**

Embracing and celebrating Black identity and beauty is an essential part of nurturing self-compassion for Black women. In a world that often marginalizes or overlooks Black voices and experiences, it is crucial for Black women to affirm their worth and value from within. Embracing Black identity involves acknowledging and honoring the richness and diversity of Black culture, history, and heritage.

One way to embrace Black identity is to cultivate a sense of pride in one's roots and ancestry. This may involve learning about Black history, traditions, and contributions to society, and connecting with cultural practices and communities. By embracing their cultural identity, women can develop a strong sense of belonging and self-esteem, grounded in a deep appreciation for who they are and where they come from.

Furthermore, celebrating Black beauty involves rejecting Eurocentric beauty standards and embracing diverse representations of beauty. Black women come in all shapes, sizes, and shades, and each individual is inherently beautiful in their own unique way. By celebrating their natural features, hairstyles, and skin tones, women can challenge social norms and affirm their inherent worth and beauty.

Additionally, surrounding oneself with positive representations of Black excellence and achievement can reinforce feelings of pride and self-worth. This may involve seeking out media, literature, and artwork that celebrate Black voices and experiences, and amplifying Black voices in one's personal and professional circles. By uplifting and supporting one another, women can create a culture of celebration and empowerment that nourishes self-compassion and resilience.

## Practicing Forgiveness and Letting Go of Guilt

Practicing forgiveness and letting go of guilt is another essential aspect of nurturing self-compassion for Black women. Oftentimes, women carry the weight of intergenerational trauma, systemic oppression, and societal expectations, which can manifest as feelings of guilt, shame, and unworthiness. Learning to forgive oneself and others is a powerful practice that can free Black women from the burdens of the past and cultivate inner peace and healing.

Forgiveness involves releasing resentment, anger, and bitterness towards oneself and others, and choosing to extend compassion and understanding instead. This can be a challenging process, especially when faced with deep-seated pain and betrayal. However, by recognizing that holding onto grudges only perpetuates suffering, Black women can begin to let go of the past and create space for healing and growth.

Moreover, forgiving oneself is an essential part of self-compassion. women may struggle with feelings of inadequacy or self-blame due to social pressures and expectations. However, it is important to recognize that everyone makes mistakes and experiences setbacks, and that failure is a natural part of the human experience. By practicing self-forgiveness, women can cultivate a sense of self-acceptance and worthiness, regardless of past actions or shortcomings.

Nurturing self-compassion involves embracing and celebrating Black identity and beauty, and practicing forgiveness and letting go of guilt. By affirming their inherent worth and value, and releasing the burdens of the past, women can cultivate a deep sense of self-compassion and resilience that sustains them in their journey towards emotional well-being and fulfillment.

# Building Supportive Relationships

Building supportive relationships is vital for emotional self-care, providing women with the necessary network of love, understanding, and empowerment. In this section, we explore two key aspects of fostering supportive relationships: navigating friendships, family dynamics, and community support, and setting boundaries and advocating for your needs.

**Navigating Friendships, Family Dynamics, and Community Support**
Navigating relationships with friends, family, and community members can significantly impact a woman's emotional well-being. Cultivating supportive friendships with individuals who uplift, validate, and understand one's experiences is essential for fostering a sense of belonging and connection. Surrounding oneself with a diverse and inclusive community that

celebrates diversity and empowers its members can provide a valuable source of strength and resilience.

In addition to friendships, navigating family dynamics can present unique challenges and opportunities for growth. women may experience tensions or conflicts within their families due to differences in values, beliefs, or generational perspectives. However, maintaining open and honest communication, setting healthy boundaries, and practicing empathy and understanding can help navigate these challenges and strengthen family bonds.

Moreover, seeking support from community organizations, cultural groups, or spiritual communities can provide additional sources of support and validation. Engaging in activities and initiatives that align with one's values and interests can foster a sense of belonging and purpose, while also connecting with like-minded individuals who share similar experiences and aspirations.

## Setting Boundaries and Advocating for Your Needs

Setting boundaries and advocating for one's needs is crucial for maintaining healthy and fulfilling relationships. women often face the expectation to be strong, self-sacrificing, and endlessly supportive, which can lead to burnout and resentment if their own needs are consistently overlooked or disregarded.

Setting boundaries involves clearly communicating one's limits, preferences, and expectations in relationships and advocating for oneself assertively. This may involve saying no to requests or demands that exceed one's capacity, expressing discomfort or dissatisfaction with certain behaviors or interactions, and prioritizing self-care and well-being.

Furthermore, advocating for one's needs involves recognizing and valuing one's worth and contributions, and asserting oneself in spaces where one's voice and experiences may be marginalized or silenced. This may involve advocating for equal opportunities and representation, challenging discriminatory practices or policies, and advocating for systemic change that benefits women and communities.

In conclusion, building supportive relationships involves navigating friendships, family dynamics, and community support, and setting boundaries and advocating for one's needs. By cultivating relationships that uplift, validate, and empower, and advocating for oneself assertively and confidently, Black women can create a network of support and validation that sustains them in their journey towards emotional well-being and fulfillment.

# Coping with Stress and Anxiety

Stress and anxiety are common experiences for many individuals, and Black women, in particular, may face unique stressors due to systemic racism, gender discrimination, and societal pressures. Coping with stress and anxiety is essential for maintaining emotional well-being and resilience. In this section, we explore strategies for managing daily stressors and addressing anxiety and panic attacks.

**Strategies for Managing Daily Stressors**
Managing daily stressors is crucial for preventing chronic stress and its negative effects on physical and emotional health. Black women may encounter a variety of stressors in their daily lives, including work pressures, family responsibilities, financial concerns, and societal injustices. Implementing effective stress management

strategies can help alleviate tension and promote a sense of calm and balance.

One strategy for managing daily stressors is to prioritize self-care activities that promote relaxation and rejuvenation. This may include engaging in regular exercise, practicing mindfulness meditation, or enjoying hobbies and activities that bring joy and fulfillment. Taking breaks throughout the day to recharge and reset can help prevent burnout and increase resilience in the face of stressors.

Additionally, developing healthy coping mechanisms for dealing with stress is essential. This may involve seeking social support from friends, family, or support groups, expressing emotions through creative outlets such as writing or art, or practicing relaxation techniques such as deep breathing or progressive muscle relaxation. By developing a toolkit of coping strategies, women can effectively navigate daily stressors and build resilience over time.

Furthermore, cultivating a supportive environment at home and in the workplace can help mitigate stressors and create a sense of safety and belonging. This may involve setting boundaries with toxic individuals, advocating for one's needs and rights, and seeking out inclusive spaces that value diversity and equity. Building a strong support network of trusted individuals who offer validation, encouragement, and practical assistance can provide a buffer against stress and promote emotional well-being.

**Addressing Anxiety and Panic Attacks**
Anxiety and panic attacks can be overwhelming experiences that disrupt daily life and cause significant distress. Black women may be particularly vulnerable to anxiety due to systemic injustices, racial trauma, and societal expectations. Addressing anxiety and panic attacks

involves implementing coping strategies to manage symptoms and seeking professional support when needed.

One effective strategy for addressing anxiety is to practice relaxation techniques that promote a sense of calm and relaxation. This may include deep breathing exercises, progressive muscle relaxation, or guided imagery. By practicing these techniques regularly, women can reduce the intensity of anxiety symptoms and regain a sense of control over the air emotions.

Moreover, challenging negative thought patterns and cognitive distortions is essential for managing anxiety. women may experience internalized racism or negative self-talk that exacerbates feelings of anxiety and self-doubt. By identifying and challenging these distorted thoughts, individuals can reframe their perspectives and develop more balanced and realistic interpretations of themselves and their experiences.

Additionally, seeking professional support from a therapist or counselor can provide valuable tools and techniques for managing anxiety and panic attacks. Cognitive-behavioral therapy (CBT) is particularly effective for treating anxiety disorders, as it helps individuals identify and modify maladaptive thought patterns and behaviors. Therapy can also provide a safe and supportive space for processing difficult emotions, exploring underlying trauma, and developing coping strategies tailored to individual needs.

Coping with stress and anxiety is essential for maintaining emotional well-being and resilience. By implementing strategies for managing daily stressors and addressing anxiety and panic attacks, women can cultivate a sense of calm, balance, and empowerment in their lives. Seeking support from trusted individuals and professionals can provide additional resources and guidance for navigating challenges and promoting overall well-being.

# Healing from Trauma

Trauma, whether historical or interpersonal, can have profound and lasting effects on an individual's emotional well-being. For Black women, the legacy of systemic racism, gender discrimination, and intergenerational trauma can manifest in various forms of psychological distress. Healing from trauma involves understanding its roots, seeking professional help and therapy, and engaging in self-care practices that promote healing and resilience.

## Understanding Historical and Interpersonal Trauma

Historical trauma refers to the cumulative emotional and psychological wounds experienced by individuals or communities as a result of systemic oppression, colonization, slavery, or other forms of historical injustice. For Black women, historical trauma encompasses the enduring impact of slavery, segregation, and ongoing racial discrimination on mental health and well-being. This includes the transmission of trauma across generations, as well as the normalization of violence, injustice, and inequality within society.

Interpersonal trauma, on the other hand, refer to traumatic experiences that occur within personal relationships, such as physical or sexual abuse, domestic violence, or childhood neglect. Black women may be disproportionately affected by interpersonal trauma due to intersecting factors such as race, gender, and socioeconomic status. Additionally, the intersectionality of oppression can increase the effects of trauma, leading to complex and intersecting forms of psychological distress.

Understanding the roots of historical and interpersonal trauma is essential for healing, as it provides context for the experiences and emotions that arise. Recognizing the impact of systemic injustice and discrimination on mental health allows individuals to validate their experiences, connect with others who share similar struggles, and advocate for systemic change.

**Seeking Professional Help and Therapy**
Seeking professional help and therapy is a crucial step in healing from trauma and reclaiming one's sense of agency and well-being. Therapy provides a safe and confidential space for individuals to explore their experiences, process difficult emotions, and develop coping strategies for managing symptoms of trauma.

There are various therapeutic approaches that can be effective in addressing trauma, including cognitive-behavioral therapy (CBT), dialectical behavior therapy (DBT), eye movement desensitization and reprocessing (EMDR), and trauma-informed therapy. These approaches focus on helping individuals understand the connection between their thoughts, emotions, and behaviors, and develop skills for regulating emotions, managing triggers, and building resilience.

Additionally, culturally competent therapy is essential for Black women seeking support for trauma-related issues. Culturally competent therapists understand the unique cultural, social, and historical contexts that shape women's experiences of trauma and can provide culturally relevant interventions and support. This may include incorporating Afrocentric perspectives, rituals, and traditions into therapy, and addressing issues of race, identity, and empowerment within the therapeutic process.

Furthermore, group therapy and support groups can be valuable resources for individuals healing from trauma. Connecting with others who have experienced similar challenges can reduce feelings of isolation and shame, provide validation and understanding, and offer opportunities for mutual support and growth. Group therapy allows individuals to share their experiences, learn from others' perspectives, and practice new coping skills in a supportive and empathetic environment.

Healing from trauma involves understanding the roots of historical and interpersonal trauma, seeking professional help and therapy, and engaging in self-care practices that promote healing and resilience. By acknowledging the impact of trauma on mental health, accessing culturally competent support, and connecting with others who share similar experiences, women can reclaim their sense of agency and well-being and embark on a journey of healing and empowerment.

# Embracing Resilience and Empowerment

Embracing resilience and empowerment is essential for you, as a woman, navigating the myriad challenges and adversities you may encounter in life. Resilience involves your ability to bounce back from setbacks, adapt to change, and thrive in the face of adversity. Empowerment, on the other hand, is about recognizing your worth, agency, and ability to effect positive change in your life and community. In this section, we explore two key aspects of embracing resilience and empowerment for you: drawing strength from your cultural heritage and resilience, and cultivating confidence and assertiveness.

## Drawing Strength from Cultural Heritage and Resilience

As a woman, you have a rich cultural heritage and history of resilience that can serve as a source of strength and inspiration in challenging times. Drawing on the wisdom, traditions, and resilience of your ancestors, you can cultivate a sense of pride, identity, and belonging that sustains you through adversity.

One way to draw strength from your culture is to learn about and celebrate Black history, achievements, and contributions to society. Explore the achievements of women leaders, artists, activists, and innovators, and recognize their resilience in the face of systemic oppression and adversity. By connecting with the stories and experiences of your ancestors, you can find inspiration and validation for your own struggles and triumphs.

Furthermore, participating in cultural practices and traditions can provide a sense of connection and grounding in times of stress or uncertainty. Attend cultural events, festivals, or ceremonies, practice rituals such as storytelling, music, or dance, and connect with spiritual or religious traditions that resonate with your beliefs and values. By engaging with cultural heritage in meaningful ways, you can cultivate a sense of belonging and empowerment that strengthens your resilience and sense of identity.

Moreover, building support networks within the Black community can provide valuable resources and solidarity in times of need. Connect with other women who share similar experiences and values to share wisdom, offer mutual support, and advocate for collective empowerment and social change. By standing together in solidarity, you can amplify your voices, challenge systemic injustices, and create a more equitable and inclusive society for future generations.

**Cultivating Confidence and Assertiveness**

Cultivating confidence and assertiveness is essential for you, as a woman, to navigate challenges, pursue your goals, and advocate for your needs and rights. Confidence involves believing in your abilities, worth, and potential, while assertiveness involves expressing yourself confidently and respectfully, advocating for your needs and boundaries, and standing up for yourself in the face of adversity.

One way to cultivate confidence is to challenge self-limiting beliefs and negative self-talk that undermine your sense of self-worth and potential. You may internalize social messages that perpetuate stereotypes, imposter syndrome, or feelings of inadequacy. By recognizing these beliefs as false and reframing them with affirming and empowering statements, you can cultivate a more positive and resilient mindset.

Furthermore, setting and achieving goals, no matter how small, can build confidence and self-efficacy over time. Break goals down into manageable steps, celebrate progress, and learn from setbacks. By doing so, you can develop a sense of competence and mastery that bolsters your confidence and resilience.

Additionally, practicing assertiveness involves expressing yourself confidently and respectfully in interpersonal interactions, setting healthy boundaries, and advocating for your needs and rights. You may face unique challenges in asserting yourself due to societal expectations, stereotypes, or fears of backlash or rejection. However, assertiveness is a skill that can be learned and practiced over time through assertiveness training, role-playing exercises, and setting small, achievable goals for assertive behavior.

In conclusion, embracing resilience and empowerment involves drawing strength from your cultural heritage and resilience, and cultivating confidence and assertiveness. By connecting with the wisdom and resilience of your ancestors, building supportive networks within the Black community, and challenging self-limiting beliefs, you can cultivate a sense of pride, identity, and agency that sustains you through adversity and empowers you to create positive change in your life and community.

# Practicing Self-Care Rituals

Practicing self-care rituals is essential for you, as a woman, to prioritize your well-being and nourish your mind, body, and spirit. Self-care involves intentionally setting aside time and space to nurture yourself, recharge your energy, and cultivate a sense of balance and harmony in your life. In this section, we explore two key aspects of practicing self-care rituals: incorporating physical, mental, and spiritual practices, and creating a personalized self-care routine that meets your unique needs and preferences.

## Incorporating Physical, Mental, and Spiritual Practices

Incorporating physical, mental, and spiritual practices into your self-care routine allows you to address your holistic well-being and cultivate a sense of wholeness and vitality.

**-Physical Practices:** Physical self-care involves taking care of your body through movement, nourishment, and rest. Engage in regular exercise that you enjoy, whether it's yoga, dancing, or going for a walk in nature. Prioritize nourishing your body with nutritious foods that fuel your energy and support your overall health. Make sure to also prioritize rest and relaxation, getting enough sleep each night and taking breaks throughout the day to recharge.

-**Mental Practices:** Mental self-care involves nurturing your mind and emotions, reducing stress, and promoting mental clarity and resilience. Practice mindfulness meditation to cultivate present moment awareness and reduce anxiety and stress. Engage in activities that stimulate your mind and creativity, such as reading, journaling, or solving puzzles. Set boundaries with technology and social media to protect your mental spaces and focus on activities that bring you joy and fulfillment.

-**Spiritual Practices:** Spiritual self-care involves connecting with your inner wisdom, purpose, and sense of meaning and belonging. Engage in spiritual practices that resonate with your beliefs and values, whether it's prayer, meditation, or spending time in nature. Connect with your spiritual community or seek out spiritual mentors and guides who can support you on your journey of self-discovery and growth. Cultivate gratitude and appreciation for the blessings in your life, fostering a sense of abundance and fulfillment.

## Creating a Personalized Self-Care Routine

Creating a personalized self-care routine allows you to tailor your self-care practices to meet your unique needs, preferences, and lifestyle. By intentionally designing a routine that supports your well-being, you can cultivate greater resilience, vitality, and joy in your life.

**-Identify Your Needs:** Start by reflecting on your current lifestyle and identifying areas where you could benefit from more self-care. Are you feeling physically exhausted and in need of more rest? Are you experiencing high levels of stress and anxiety and in need of more mental self-care? Are you feeling disconnected from your spiritual practice and in need of more spiritual nourishment? Take stock of your needs and priorities to guide your self-care routine.

**-Set Realistic Goals:** Set realistic and achievable goals for your self-care routine, taking into account your schedule, resources, and energy levels. Start small and gradually build momentum over time, adding new practices or rituals as you feel ready. Be gentle and compassionate with yourself, recognizing that self-care is an ongoing journey of discovery and growth.

**-Experiment and Explore:** Take time to experiment with different self-care practices and rituals to see what resonates with you. Be open to trying new activities and approaches, even if they may seem outside of your comfort zone at first. Pay attention to how each practice makes you feel and whether it brings you a sense of nourishment, joy, and fulfillment.

**-Prioritize Consistency:** Consistency is key when it comes to practicing self-care. Set aside dedicated time each day or week to engage in your self-care rituals, making them a non-negotiable part of your routine. Consider creating a self-care schedule or planner to help you stay organized and accountable to your self-care goals.

**-Listen to Your Intuition:** Trust your intuition and listen to your body's cues to guide your self-care routine. Pay attention to what feels nourishing and replenishing for you, and honor your needs and boundaries accordingly. Be flexible and adaptable, adjusting your self-care practices as needed based on changes in your circumstances or priorities.

In conclusion, practicing self-care rituals is essential for prioritizing your well-being and nourishing your mind, body, and spirit as a woman. By incorporating physical, mental, and spiritual practices into your routine and creating a personalized self-care routine that meets your unique needs and preferences, you can cultivate greater resilience, vitality, and joy in your life. Remember to be gentle and compassionate with yourself along the way, honoring your journey of self-discovery and growth.

# Balancing Work, Life, and Activism

Balancing work, life, and activism is essential for you, as a woman, to maintain your well-being, pursue your goals, and contribute to positive change in your community and society. Juggling the demands of your career, personal life, and activism can be challenging, but with intentionality and self-care, you can find harmony and fulfillment in all areas of your life. In this section, we explore two key aspects of balancing work, life, and activism: managing career goals and responsibilities, and engaging in social justice and activism while protecting your mental health.

## Managing Career Goals and Responsibilities

As a woman, managing your career goals and responsibilities requires careful planning, prioritization, and boundary-setting to ensure that you can pursue your professional aspirations while also maintaining a healthy work-life balance.

**-Set Clear Goals:** Start by setting clear and achievable goals that align with your values, interests, and strengths. Whether you aspire to advance in your current role, switch careers, or pursue entrepreneurship, having a clear vision of what you want to achieve can help guide your actions and decisions.

**-Prioritize Self-Care:** Prioritize self-care practices that nourish your mind, body, and spirit, even amidst the demands of your career. Make time for regular exercise, rest, and relaxation to recharge your energy and prevent burnout. Set boundaries with work to protect your personal time and maintain a healthy work-life balance.

**-Seek Support and Mentorship:** Seek support and mentorship from colleagues, mentors, or professional networks to help you navigate your career journey. Surround yourself with people who believe in your potential and can offer guidance, encouragement, and opportunities for growth.

**-Advocate for Yourself:** Advocate for yourself in the workplace by speaking up for your needs, interests, and aspirations. Negotiate for fair compensation, opportunities for advancement, and accommodations that support your well-being and success. Don't be afraid to assert yourself and advocate for your worth and value as a woman in the workplace.

## Engaging in Social Justice and Activism While Protecting Mental Health

Engaging in social justice and activism is a powerful way for you, as a woman, to advocate for equality, justice, and positive change in your community and society. However, it's important to prioritize your mental health and well-being while engaging in activism to prevent burnout and sustain your long-term commitment to social justice.

**-Set Boundaries:** Set boundaries around your activism work to protect your mental health and prevent overwhelm. Establish limits on the amount of time and energy you dedicate to activism, and prioritize self-care practices that replenish your energy and prevent burnout.

**-Practice Self-Compassion:** Practice self-compassion and self-care to nurture your emotional well-being amidst the challenges of activism work. Acknowledge your limitations and vulnerabilities, and be gentle and understanding with yourself when you experience setbacks or difficulties.

**-Seek Support:** Seek support from fellow activists, friends, family members, or mental health professionals when you need it. Surround yourself with a supportive community that understands the unique challenges of activism and can offer empathy, validation, and encouragement.

**-Take Breaks:** Take breaks from activism work when you need to recharge and replenish your energy. Engage in activities that bring you joy and relaxation, whether it's spending time with loved ones, pursuing hobbies, or enjoying nature.

**-Focus on Impact:** Focus on the impact and significance of your activism work, rather than getting bogged down by perfectionism or unrealistic expectations. Celebrate your successes and milestones along the way, and recognize the contributions you're making to positive change in your community and society.

Balancing work, life, and activism is essential for you, as a woman, to maintain your well-being, pursue your goals, and contribute to positive change in your community and society. By managing your career goals and responsibilities with intentionality and self-care, and engaging in social justice and activism while prioritizing your mental health, you can find harmony and fulfillment in all areas of your life. Remember to set boundaries, practice self-compassion, seek support when needed, and celebrate your contributions to positive change along the way.

# Conclusion

As you reach the end of this journey exploring emotional self-care for Black women, take a moment to reflect on your progress and growth, and reaffirm your commitment to your ongoing emotional well-being.

**Reflecting on Progress and Growth**

Throughout this exploration, you've delved into various aspects of emotional self-care, from understanding the importance of resilience and empowerment to practicing self-care rituals and balancing work, life, and activism. You've taken steps to draw strength from your cultural heritage, cultivate confidence and assertiveness, and engage in social justice and activism while protecting your mental health. Along the way, you've confronted challenges, embraced resilience, and celebrated your victories, both big and small.

Reflect on how far you've come on your journey of emotional self-care. Consider the insights you've gained, the habits you've cultivated, and the barriers you've overcome. Celebrate your growth and resilience, acknowledging the progress you've made in prioritizing your well-being and nurturing your mind, body, and spirit.

## Committing to Ongoing Emotional Self-Care Journey

As you conclude this journey, recommit yourself to your ongoing emotional self-car journey. Recognize that self-care is not a destination but a lifelong practice of self-discovery, growth, and renewal. Continue to prioritize your well-being, making time for self-care rituals, setting boundaries, and seeking support when needed.

Commit to nurturing your resilience and empowerment, drawing strength from your cultural heritage and community, and advocating for your needs and rights. Embrace self-compassion and self-love, recognizing your inherent worth and value as a woman. And remember that you are not alone on this journey—surround yourself with supportive networks and allies who uplift and empower you along the way.

In closing, know that your commitment to emotional self-care is a radical act of self-love and empowerment. By prioritizing your well-being and nurturing your mind, body, and spirit, you not only transform your own life but also contribute to positive change in your community and society. Embrace the power of self-care as a tool for resilience, healing, and liberation, and continue to shine your light brightly as you navigate the journey ahead.

www.ingramcontent.com/pod-product-compliance
Lightning Source LLC
Chambersburg PA
CBHW070727260726
48660CB00007B/2752